THE
POCKET
IDIOT'S
GUIDE™ TO

a Great Upper Body

by Tom Seabourne, Ph.D.

ALPHA

A member of the Penguin Group (USA) Inc.

This book is dedicated to my father, who will always be my inspiration.

ALPHA BOOKS

Published by the Penguin Group

Penguin Group (USA) Inc., 375 Hudson Street, New York, New York 10014, U.S.A.

Penguin Group (Canada), 10 Alcorn Avenue, Toronto, Ontario, Canada M4V 3B2 (a division of Pearson Penguin Canada Inc.)

Penguin Books Ltd, 80 Strand, London WC2R 0RL, England

Penguin Ireland, 25 St Stephen's Green, Dublin 2, Ireland (a division of Penguin Books Ltd)

Penguin Group (Australia), 250 Camberwell Road, Camberwell, Victoria 3124, Australia (a division of Pearson Australia Group Pty Ltd)

Penguin Books India Pvt Ltd, 11 Community Centre, Panchsheel Park, New Delhi—110 017, India

Penguin Group (NZ), cnr Airborne and Rosedale Roads, Albany, Auckland 1310, New Zealand (a division of Pearson New Zealand Ltd)

Penguin Books (South Africa) (Pty) Ltd, 24 Sturdee Avenue, Rosebank, Johannesburg 2196, South Africa

Penguin Books Ltd, Registered Offices: 80 Strand, London WC2R 0RL, England

International Standard Book Number: 1-59257-442-4
Library of Congress Catalog Card Number: 2005932769

07 06 05   8 7 6 5 4 3 2 1

Interpretation of the printing code: The rightmost number of the first series of numbers is the year of the book's printing; the rightmost number of the second series of numbers is the number of the book's printing. For example, a printing code of 05-1 shows that the first printing occurred in 2005.

Printed in the United States of America

Note: This publication contains the opinions and ideas of its author. It is intended to provide helpful and informative material on the subject matter covered. It is sold with the understanding that the author and publisher are not engaged in rendering professional services in the book. If the reader requires personal assistance or advice, a competent professional should be consulted.

The author and publisher specifically disclaim any responsibility for any liability, loss, or risk, personal or otherwise, which is incurred as a consequence, directly or indirectly, of the use and application of any of the contents of this book.

Most Alpha books are available at special quantity discounts for bulk purchases for sales promotions, premiums, fund-raising, or educational use. Special books, or book excerpts, can also be created to fit specific needs.

For details, write: Special Markets, Alpha Books, 375 Hudson Street, New York, NY 10014.

Contents

Appendix

Introduction

It's hard to take your eyes off of a well-developed upper body. A well-defined chest is balanced by a great-looking back to complete your upper-body package. Having great arms isn't everything, but if your shoulders are equally great-looking, you have it all.

You need three ingredients for a great upper body—the motivation to work out, an eating plan to get you cut and defined, and the best upper-body workout in existence. Whether you train in your office, at home, or in your gym, I give you the tools to get a great workout.

Your body is only going to take you so far. When the mind and body work together, you can produce better results than you ever dreamed possible. The most common excuse I hear is that people don't have time to work out. I explain how to schedule your workout into your day. My program is filled with motivational strategies to get that upper body you thought was unattainable.

With fast food and processed packaged meals around every corner, it's hard to know what to eat. The eating program is healthy, tasty, balanced, simple—and it works. My eating program is not one-size-fits-all. Instead, I individualize the foods and the meal plan to fit your lifestyle. You learn to eat when you're hungry and fuel your muscles at the appropriate times. The eating program reduces inches no matter where you carry them. I tailor the program to your needs, based on the foods you like and when you want to eat them.

I help you contour your entire upper body using a variety of exercises. My tried-and-true upper-body workout equalizes size and strength between all of your major muscle groups. Upper- and mid-back exercises are balanced with chest training. The fronts of your upper arms (biceps) and backs of your upper arms (triceps) get equal attention. And all three areas of your shoulders—front, side, and back—may be sculpted according to how you want them to look.

You can train at home, in your office, and in the gym. No muscle group is untouched; from those flabby triceps to your often-neglected upper back. If you're already doing *The Pocket Idiot's Guide to Great Abs,* you can cross-train with our upper-body–toning workouts to create an exquisite physique. We teach you to develop sleek, tight, and sexy muscles. It's not about grunting and groaning. My program is efficient and user-friendly.

You only need to do a couple of upper-body workouts a week. You will own toned arms, a V-shaped back, and well-shaped shoulders. Won't it be fun to wear sleeveless tops or low-back dresses? Feeling stronger and looking toned boosts your confidence.

If your schedule requires you to work out two days in a row, you can split up your routine. You can do upper body one day and lower body the next, with *The Pocket Idiot's Guide to Great Buns and Thighs.* Or you can train your upper body two days in a row by doing your pulling muscles (back, biceps) for one session and pushing muscles (shoulder, chest, triceps) the next.

Your exercise program doesn't require you to huff and puff. Instead, bump up your normal activities. A walk to your mailbox is as much a part of the program as lifting weights. You don't have to join a gym, but if you already belong to one, we will show you how to train. Grunting and groaning and sweating bullets will get you there, but there is another way.

In this book you will find sidebars that are tidbits of important and useful information to keep you making progress on the program.

Bet You Didn't Know

This sidebar warns you of common myths and misconceptions concerning diet and exercise.

Get It Right

This sidebar provides you with cautionary warnings to be sure you're doing your exercises right.

In Other Words

This sidebar helps you to understand the anatomy of your upper body and figure out technical or unusual terms and concepts found in the main text. For example, rhomboids, pectoralis major, latissimus dorsi, deltoids ....

Your Personal Trainer

This sidebar provides you with quick tips about how to do your exercises correctly and information to keep your form perfect.

Acknowledgments

I want to thank the photographer, Ron Barker, and our fabulous models, Brittany and Brandon. Thanks to Paul Dinas, who had the confidence in me to pursue this project, and his amazing coaching along the way. My wife, Danese, and five beautiful children, Alaina, Grant, Laura, Susanna, and Julia, are always finding new ways to make workouts fun. And finally to my brother, Rick, my sister, Barb, and my mother, Ann, who, in my opinion, own the finest fitness facility in northeastern Pennsylvania.

Special Thanks to the Technical Reviewer

The Pocket Idiot's Guide to a Great Upper Body was reviewed by an expert who double-checked the accuracy of what you'll learn here, to help us ensure that this book gives you everything you need to know. Special thanks are extended to Shannon Loveless.

Trademarks

All terms mentioned in this book that are known to be or are suspected of being trademarks or service marks have been appropriately capitalized. Alpha Books and Penguin Group (USA) Inc. cannot attest to the accuracy of this information. Use of a term in this book should not be regarded as affecting the validity of any trademark or service mark.

Chapter 1

Upper Body Made Simple

In This Chapter

- Farewell to skinny arms
- Popping pecs can be yours
- Boulder shoulders are not a dream

Ever notice someone with a great upper body walking through the mall? Your eyes are drawn to well-defined arms, a broad chest, and a tapered, V-shaped back.

Changing the shape of your upper body isn't brain surgery. Evaluate your upper body in a mirror. Decide if you want to shape and slenderize your arms and shoulders, lift up that chest, and firm your back. Be specific about the changes you would like to make according to the anatomy presented in this chapter.

Males usually want to increase the size and density of their upper body muscles. It's hard to find a man who doesn't want a big chest and sinewy arms. Women prefer an athletic, shapely, firm, and feminine body.

A well-proportioned, sleek, defined upper body is ideal.

Good genes may provide you with a great figure, but you have to earn defined muscles. The purpose of this chapter is to help you design the ideal shape for your upper body. Sure, genetics play a role, but you can improve each of your upper-body muscle groups, increase the separation between each muscle, and enhance the detail of your entire upper body.

Get It Right

There are three basic body types—endomorph, a heavy, rounded appearance; ectomorph, very thin; and mesomorph, V-shaped and muscular. Although you cannot change the shape of your muscles, sculpt them to create the best-shaped upper body your genetic potential will allow.

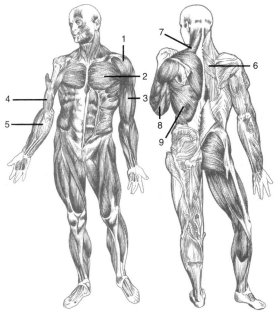

1. Deltoid (shoulder)
2. Pectoralis major (chest)
3. Biceps brachii (front upper arm)
4. Brachialis (side upper arm)
5. Brachioradialis (upper arm and forearm)

6. Rhomboids (middle back)
7. Trapezius (upper shoulder)
8. Triceps brachii (back upper arm)
9. Latissimus dorsi (upper back)

The muscle groups in your upper body.

Arms

The upper arms consist of two muscle groups, the biceps and the triceps. The biceps run along the front of the upper arms and are responsible for bending the elbow. The triceps run along the back of the arm.

Biceps

When it comes to arm training, men have an obsession with the biceps. To be able to fold up your sleeves and display peaked, rock hard, striated upper arms, is one of the greatest sensations of the male ego. Men want big biceps because they are visible in the mirror and attract the attention of others—not just from the opposite sex, but also among their peers.

Make a muscle by bending your elbow and bringing your fist toward your shoulder. The biceps consist of an inner and outer head on the top side of your upper arm. The *biceps brachii* is your beach muscle. Although some people can make this muscle peak at the top when they flex it, genetics plays a huge role in the actual shape of the muscle.

The *brachialis muscle* is underneath your biceps and adds fullness to your arm. You can see this muscle better from a side view.

Your Personal Trainer _____

Spend more time focusing your training on your major muscle groups (chest, back, and shoulders) instead of worrying about your arms. When you train your large muscle groups, your arms are working, too.

Triceps

Women are concerned less about the size of their biceps and more about firmness and definition. The focal point of female upper-arm training is the triceps in the back of the arm.

Well-defined triceps are very attractive. A toned set of triceps creates an image of youth, vitality, and sexiness. Everyone wants to bare his or her arms and be buffed and tank top–ready. Well-toned triceps are a perfect warm-weather accessory. With a little effort, sculpted triceps are within your reach.

The triceps run along the back of the upper arm. Their purpose is to extend the elbow to straighten the arm. Your triceps muscles are almost double the size of your biceps.

The triceps are two thirds of the muscle mass of your upper arms. Since your triceps has three heads and your biceps only two, your biceps will never catch up to your triceps; nor should they.

Extend your elbows to the front with your palms facing down. Find a mirror and look at the back of your upper arms. Your defined triceps are shaped like miniature horseshoes.

Back

One of the first mistakes people make when training the upper body is to train the muscles they can see—chest and arms. Your chest and arms are small muscle groups compared to your back. They don't have as much potential for adding a visual change to your body.

The back muscles are neglected because you don't see them every day, but your back is important in creating an overall symmetrical physique that is pleasing to the eye. Women want a toned back because it helps them to stand taller and stop that nagging bra-strap bulge. A V-back silhouette gives the appearance of a narrow waist and smaller hips, as well as creating the illusion that your arms are more developed.

Feel the widest part of your back just behind your armpit. Those are your *latissimus dorsi* muscles, or lats. The lats are the largest back muscle, and the ones that give most of the "V-taper" to your upper body. Your lats run the entire length of your back from your shoulders to your hips. Well-toned lats add shape and width to your upper body. A lat spread that fans out resembles a cobra's head. If you develop your lats, your friends will notice immediately.

Another important set of back muscles is the *rhomboids.* These are small rectangular muscles at the center of your back just beneath your shoulders. They are named after the geometric parallelogram with no right angles and adjacent sides of unequal length. They have two parts, a major and minor, and are located on both sides of the upper part of your spine.

If you work at a desk all day, you probably round your back. Sloppy posture is unattractive. Pull your shoulders back and down. Your rhomboids are the muscles that did most of the work. A poised, confident look is important. Your rhomboids are one of the major muscle groups responsible for maintaining perfect upper-body posture. Flex your rhomboids and your shoulders stay back and your chest naturally extends outward. Your rhomboids counteract the tendency to hunch your shoulders. You feel better and look better with strong, toned rhomboids.

Shoulders

Whether you're fat or thin, dressed for work or for the beach, wide shoulders give a powerful impression. Broad shoulders are the most visible part of your "X-frame." Your shoulders are the top of the "V" created by your sleek back. Great-looking shoulders hide possible flaws in your waist and the rest of your upper body. Broad shoulders combined with a V-back create the illusion of a smaller waist, even if your waist size doesn't change.

To see just how much of a difference this makes, take a pair of socks and stuff them inside your shirt on each side of your shoulders. Then look in the mirror. Even a small increase in width completely transforms your appearance.

In Other Words

You have four rotator cuff muscles that attach your shoulder to your upper arm bone. They are your supraspinatus, infraspinatus, teres minor, and subscapularis.

Shapely shoulders can be yours with a little effort. Cup your right hand on your left shoulder. Raise your left hand toward the ceiling and you can feel your shoulder muscles flex. Any pressing movement over your head involves your shoulders.

Your shoulder muscles, or *deltoids*, have three parts— *medial*, *anterior*, and *posterior*. Feel your medial deltoids by raising your arms from your sides as if you were doing slow-motion jumping jacks. This is the muscle that widens your X-frame, and, if you train hard enough, will make the sides of your shoulders the size of softballs.

Flex the front of your shoulder (anterior deltoid) by raising your arm to the front. The anterior deltoid muscles are visible just to the outside of your chest muscles. When these muscles are defined, it's hard to take your eyes off of them.

Don't forget to train the back of your shoulder (posterior deltoid). The posterior deltoids look awesome when they are cut and defined. They are located further back on your shoulder, just above your shoulder blade. These muscles make an impression when someone sees you from behind.

Traps

It is important for you to identify each set of shoulder muscles so you can increase them, tone them, or leave them alone. You have a nice-sized chest, well-defined delts, and your lats are so wide your elbows don't touch your sides anymore. But the mirror tells you that something is missing. Your head and neck don't seem to have a solid base of support.

This is where your *trapezius* (traps) comes in. Your traps are a set of muscles that are often overlooked, because they're not in your immediate vision. You don't recognize them as a separate muscle because you use them when you train almost every other upper-body part.

Your traps are thick, triangular muscles that run from your neck across the top of the shoulder, and down along your backbone to the middle of your back. These kite-shaped muscles are the largest muscle group in your upper shoulder. A toned set of traps adds shape to your shoulders and upper back.

Use your traps to shrug your shoulders. Your traps also work with your deltoids to raise your hand. If your traps become too large you might begin to resemble a cartoon character.

 Bet You Didn't Know _____

> If a muscle becomes too large, stop training it. If a muscle is not used, it atrophies. Use it or lose it.

Chest

A wimpy chest detracts from an impressive upper body. An undefined chest makes you look older than your years. A sculpted chest appears attractive even if your lower body carries more fat than it should.

A broad chest is perhaps the most widely sought muscle group of the human physique. It is rare to find a gym goer, particularly a male, who isn't looking to put another inch or two on the chest. It is the body part that even skinny guys on the beach try to develop.

Place your right hand on your left chest muscle. Push your desk with your left hand. Feel the chest muscles stimulated by the pushing movement. Now place your right hand on your left chest muscle. This time, move your left arm horizontally, back and forth. Your chest muscles flex when you bring your arm toward the middle of your body.

Ideal chest development is not a hanging, bulbous mass, but muscles that are fully defined from top to bottom. The chest muscles run all the way from your collarbone to just below your nipple.

For guys with low body fat, the chest muscles cut a sharp, flaring line clearly delineating the outer and lower chest border. The chest muscles are fan-shaped, and the outer and lower fibers are one and the same muscle.

Your chest muscles are referred to as pectoral muscles. The *pectoralis major* can be felt under the breast when the muscle is flexed. The *pectoralis minor* is near your collarbone on the upper chest.

The pectoralis major is larger and attaches to the sternum. The pectoralis minor connects to the collarbone. Both pectoralis muscles are surrounded by the collarbone, sternum, and rib cage, and are attached to the upper-arm bone.

Chapter 2

Give Me Ten!

In This Chapter

- The right day, the right time
- Seeing is believing
- Mind over muscle
- Get started, it's now or never

Congratulations, purchasing this book is your most important step in getting a toned upper body. Choose your goal—having a well-developed chest, or just being able to wear a sleeveless tee shirt; adding an inch of muscle to your chest in two months; or taking an inch of flab off your arms. Quick goals keep you pumped up for the long haul. Don't compare your progress to others; it takes as long as it takes for you.

Take a minute and think about what you will look like in a bathing suit after a couple months of working out. It will feel great to have an upper body you can be proud of. Pull your shoulders back and sit up tall knowing that your shapely shoulders are just around the corner. Don't just read this sentence.

Create a detailed mental picture of your defined chest and arms. Find a picture of a person you admire or would like to look like with your same body structure to motivate you.

Brain Training Is Key

A quick examination of how your goals and desires fit your personality can go a long way toward helping you stay with your exercise program. You may prefer to work out at home, in the office, in a gym, or all of the above. Your personality may lead you to a strict regimen, or cross-training in a variety of exercises.

 Your Personal Trainer

No muscle is as hard to train as your back. Get in front of a double mirror and check out your reps so you can make the mind-to-muscle connection.

Don't just start working out. Get on a program you believe in. This will increase your motivation and provide you with the confidence to stick with your workout to deliver the results you desire.

Although you may have given up on working out in the past, this program is doable. You don't have to pick one form of exercise and plod through it for the rest of your life. Any exercise that gets you off the couch is fine.

Schedule Your Workout to Fit

Be honest. In the past, when you missed workouts or quit programs, it was partly because you were lazy. This program will help you to figure out what works for you when it comes to staying motivated for longer than a week or two.

Schedule your meals and workout into your day. The best time to work out is whenever it consistently fits into your schedule. Working out in the morning is a great way to start your day. It's an energizing way to stimulate your metabolism and there is less chance that your workout will be interrupted.

Scheduling your workout for later in the evening may be a disaster. Putting off your training until after work or dinner usually means that it won't get done. Before you know it, you will feel sleepy and it's bedtime.

Schedule your workout for a set exact time on each workout day. Be faithful to this schedule no matter what.

To get started, your favorite 30-minute easy daily activity plus a couple days of toning and stretching is all you need. Keep your workouts balanced and progressing. This will keep you motivated.

Fifty percent of those who begin an exercise program quit within the first six months because of lack of time, injury, negative emotions, poor social support, or low motivation. You can be in the successful fifty percent that faces these adversities and overcomes them.

Finding the Workout that Works

A combination of your eating program and isolation training is your blueprint for a tight, toned upper body. But you have to get started. First thing tomorrow morning, schedule your workout.

But be careful, an overzealous training schedule might be the last thing you need. Start slow and progress gradually. Choose activities you love. People who stick with their workout programs are not more disciplined than you. They simply have found a program that they look forward to doing.

Create workouts that aren't workouts. Any easy activity counts toward your exercise time. Moving around feels good and getting up and out the door gives you a break from your normal routine.

The back of your arms won't stop waving after one workout, but you will feel so much better about yourself. Your energy level will increase and you will catch yourself glancing in the mirror to check out your arms. Use the photos in this book to motivate your training. Your chest and back will flex automatically and your posture will improve. Give yourself a reasonable amount of time to notice results.

The fat around your upper back doesn't know whether you are walking or skating. And your chest muscles will firm up whether you use free weights or exercise bands. If you hate the thought of "working" out, go out and play with your kids or have fun with a sport. Push your kids on swings, or play volleyball or tennis. Different activities keep your exercise program balanced. Try new things to keep your fitness moving forward. Use muscles you haven't used before. Challenge your coordination with one-legged exercises. Try playing a game of catch with your other hand.

Most people start working out too hard or not hard enough. If you can only endure for five minutes, so be it. Add two minutes a week until you are training for 30 minutes. You don't have to work out at your target heart rate five days a week and eat like a health nut. Re-evaluate your goals so that your exercise is specific to what you really want.

If you don't have much time to work out, break up your program into manageable parts. A full half-hour may be out of the question, so separate your workout into three ten-minute segments.

Alternate five-minute bouts of easy activity with five minutes of upper body–isolation, or even five minutes of a different form of easy activity. Segmenting your workout into small chunks is fun and gives you great results in a short period of time.

Keeping a log of your workouts can help prevent overtraining or undertraining. Writing down how long you walked or how much weight you lifted is objective evidence that you are making progress.

Integrating Workouts and Life

Make your eating program and workouts a habit. Do not miss any meals or workouts for your first month. Clear your schedule to be sure there are no conflicts.

If you dread exercise and eating properly, tell yourself you can quit after a month. Reward yourself after each successful day of eating and exercise with massages, manicures, or clothing. Create short and long-term goals as well for motivational purposes.

After you have been working out for a while, instead of choosing the best "calorie burner," ask your body how the new workout makes you feel.

During your easy-activity workouts, let your mind wander. Your most creative ideas come to you when you're doing a repetitive activity that doesn't require your full concentration. But don't set out to cure cancer. Use your easy-activity time to answer less-pressing questions so your workouts don't become work.

Use your favorite tunes to pump up your efforts. Listen to whatever music gets you in the mood to move. Burn your own CDs of motivating rhythms, alternating fast and slow beats to coincide with the intensity of your workouts.

Another popular motivational training tool to measure your exercise progression is a heart rate monitor (HRM). Use an HRM to figure out if you are working out too hard or too easy. They are easy to use and are more accurate than taking your pulse from the neck or wrist. Just as your antique personal computer cost a fortune, early HRMs were pricey. Today you can pick one up for less than what you would pay for dinner and a movie.

You may be the type of person who needs to get pumped up before you work out. But being too jazzed causes you to lose focus. And if you are too relaxed, you may catch yourself reclining on the couch. Get pumped up, but not too much. Your mind affects your workout. Use music, an HRM, TV, or whatever it takes to tie those shoes and get moving.

Eating rituals are important, too. Schedule meals in advance and sit down to all of your meals. Be consistent. Discipline is a skill that improves with practice. It is better to be consistent and steady than to be perfect for a week and then quit.

Get It Right

You should feel energized and revitalized after your workout. If you feel sluggish and tired, you did too much.

You don't have to join a gym, but it sure helps. Sign up for a long-term membership so that you will be wasting your hard-earned money if you don't go. You will make new friends at the gym. Choose a friend as a training partner. Meet your partner at a specific time to work out. Training with like-minded people is motivating, a bit of healthy competition is fun, and a committment with a workout partner is difficult to break, too! The feeling of driving home from the gym with a lifted chest, toned arms, and a V-back can't be beat.

Pushing Through the Burn

Stay cool no matter what. If something goes wrong during your workout, note it, adjust, and then go on. If you don't get to all of your exercises tell yourself you will get to them next time.

Even your best-laid plans may go awry. A phone call five minutes before your workout or an unexpected trip out of town can ruin your schedule. Have a back-up plan. Reschedule your activity or take an exercise band in your suitcase for your out-of-town workout.

Change negative feelings and thoughts that distract you from your goal. Mentally prepare for an unexpected event. If the phone rings during your home workout, let the answering machine pick it up. Make fitness a priority in your life, and you will have a firm and tight upper body before you know it.

If you strain a muscle, see your physician and ask if there is a way to work around the problem. Be open to doing different activities outside of your usual regimen.

Bet You Didn't Know

If you strain a muscle in your arm or leg, don't forget about the other 75 percent of your body that is looking forward to your workout.

No matter your intentions, it's not *if* you miss a workout, it's *when*. You are not perfect in other areas of your life, and your workouts won't be perfect, either. Obsessing about exercise is worse than not exercising at all. If you feel as if you can't miss a day, you may be setting yourself up for an overuse injury. Your muscles need to rest and rejuvenate at least one day each week; your mind needs a day off too. A day off may be just what you need to attack your workout the next day. Giving yourself a mental break prevents burn-out and makes you more likely to stick to your long-term exercise program.

In Other Words

Abstinence violation is psycho-babble that means when you miss a day of your workout or eating program you decide to give up and throw in the towel.

Plan for lapses and relapses. Too many people fall off the wagon and then give up. Lapses are part of this program. Cheating on meals and an occasional week off from exercise are not only acceptable, they're required. Skip a workout on purpose to prove to yourself that falling off the wagon is no big deal. The next day, get right back on the wagon.

Add a Ritual or Consistent Routine

Before biceps curls, set your feet, bring your elbows in close, shoulders back, chest out, take a deep breath, and begin your first rep.

Don't rush through your workout. How many times have you seen gym rats (not you, of course) using their backs to swing the weights up, instead of using good form? They strain their muscles so bad they can't work out for a month.

Try this strategy to work the proper muscles and stay safe: Begin by sitting with perfect posture. Squeeze your hands into fists, relax. Bring your shoulders toward your ears, relax. Press your heels into the floor, relax. Press your lower back into the chair, relax.

This teaches you to be aware of your muscles while you are training them. Then, when you are doing your upper-body exercises, you will notice if you are unnecessarily straining other muscles.

Visualize Your Upper Body

You want to have firm arms and a streamlined back. Imagine what you will look like after a month on the program. If you think you are too tired to work out, begin your warm-up. If you still feel tired, go for an easy stroll instead of doing your full-blown power walk.

Picture the training it will take to look good in your swimsuit. When you visualize yourself training, nervous impulses are sent down pathways to stimulate muscle fibers. So you're actually getting a workout just thinking about your well-defined upper body.

Imagine performing the bench press. Pretend you are lying on your back on the bench. Pull your shoulder blades together, your feet firmly planted on the floor, and grab the steel bar. Feel your chest muscles flexing as you take the bar off of the rack and lower it toward your chest. Congratulations. You actually created a mind-to-muscle connection.

Watch a mental movie of yourself training. All elite athletes do this. Seeing your workout before you do it is not hocus-pocus; it makes your upper-body workout easier and more effective. Imagine you are in the cafeteria line. What foods will you choose?

Place your right hand on your left upper arm. Feel the definition. Imagine yourself doing a biceps curl. Feel the imaginary flexing of your arm muscles. The more you practice in your head, the more ripped and toned your arms will become.

Daydream about your goals and you'll get them. Self-talk such as "My arms are becoming defined" raises your enthusiasm. Use your sense of humor every chance you get. Keep your mind on your workout. Use emotions to pump up or relax. Feel strong and know that your body can handle the physical effort. Remain confident no matter what.

Chapter 3

Beyond Reps

In This Chapter

- Less is best—don't overtrain
- Keep your chest up
- Upper body: firm, toned, and strong
- High-definition principles

A toned upper body makes a lasting first impression. A streamlined back, rounded shoulders, a broad chest, and defined arms can be yours with a little planning and hard work. All you need is a few minutes a day, three days a week. Combine my upper-body exercise program with a smart eating plan, and you will see visible results in a month.

Toning your back and shoulders doesn't just happen in the gym. Normal household activities can improve the definition in your upper body. Hold a watermelon in your arms. Muscles in your back must counterbalance it. Hold it next to your side. Muscles on the other side brace your effort. Whenever you push or pull, your chest, back, shoulders, and arms do the work.

Form

Keep your form perfect and maintain normal breathing. All exercises should be performed in a controlled manner and in a range of motion that is comfortable.

Maintain perfect posture on every exercise.

Keep your stomach in; relax your neck; keep your back flat (don't arch). Draw your navel in toward your spine by contracting your lower abs. Do this before and during all of your upper-body exercises.

Focus on a specific part of your upper body. For example, to train your chest, think about pushing away from your body. Relax the remainder of your body so a higher percentage of force is exerted behind the specific muscle group you are working.

Never let the amount of weight or repetitions dictate form.

If you are training the fronts of your arms, keep the backs of your arms relaxed. Grunt if you want, but the rest of your body is relaxed. Move smoothly into each repetition with a controlled and yet one hundred percent energized effort.

Move through a full range of motion on each of your upper-body exercises. Ease into your workout. Start with some easy repetitions, and then gradually increase the intensity. Breathe normally during an exercise; however, if you are exerting, exhale during the contraction. Inhale on your short rests between each contraction.

Balance is important for symmetrical development of your chest, back, shoulders, and arms. An unbalanced workout program can lead to a difference in strength between your chest, back, and shoulders. When this happens, you are more susceptible to injuries.

Muscle groups that oppose each other need to be balanced. Development between your biceps and triceps should be balanced. Fortunately, this program has built-in exercises so that you will be training all of your upper-body muscle groups.

Speed

Take your time on each repetition. The slower you move, the less momentum, and the more work your muscles are accomplishing. You should be able to stop at any point during your rep.

Three seconds in both directions works well.

During each repetition of your upper-body workout there are two different parts. One part is called the *positive* or "up" phase of the repetition. The second part is the *negative* or "down" phase of the repetition. It is important to come down slowly on the negative phase. Moving slowly on the negative phase will speed your progress to chisel that upper body.

Bet You Didn't Know

A full range of motion means to stretch each muscle group to 1.2 times its normal resting length on each rep.

Slower uses more muscle fibers.

Don't worry about how much weight or how many reps you can do. Instead, think about the quality of your movement. If you are too fatigued to do the negative portion of the rep with perfect control, then you have done enough reps for that exercise.

Your upper-body muscles will respond very well when you are using good form at a controlled speed. Cheating on your reps leads to injury. Don't try to keep up with someone else. Work at your own pace.

Resistance

Resistance training tones your upper-body muscles. Use dumbbells, bands, or your own body weight to challenge your chest, back, shoulders, and arms. Pushing and pulling doors are forms of resistance, too.

Training your upper body with resistance increases your lean muscle mass. The more lean muscle you have, the more calories your body burns. There is no better way to contour and streamline your upper body than by using resistance. You cannot spot-lose body fat, but you can tone your upper-body muscles.

Your metabolism may be defined as how many calories your body uses, even while sleeping, breathing, or reading this book. Muscle makes up about 25 percent of your metabolic rate. Muscle tissue burns more calories than fat tissue, with each pound burning about 50 calories a day. Each pound of fat only burns about 2 calories a day.

A major factor behind losing your metabolism is muscle loss. After age 25 you lose about a half-pound of muscle each year. If you don't start toning, you will lose 5 pounds of muscle and replace it with about 15 pounds of fat every decade. It's no wonder that your friends who eat the same now as they did in high school are 30 pounds overweight. Resistance training will help shrink flab on the backs of your arms. The muscle tissue firms up to speed your sluggish metabolism. Muscle is toned and more compact than fat.

Your upper-body muscles will tone and tighten in response to repetitive exercise against progressively increased resistance. As your muscles adapt to a given weight, that weight must be gradually increased to stimulate further improvement. The key to strength and muscle tone is the overload principle. Overloading involves applying a greater-than-normal stress to your upper-body muscles. The overload may be increased weight, reps, sets, or less rest between sets. Upper-body exercises that do not overload your muscles have little benefit.

Your upper body won't get muscle-bound from resistance training. Women are especially concerned that they will develop huge arms and shoulders. Since females don't have high levels of testosterone, they won't get big and bulky, if they train the right way. Even swimsuit models lift weights.

In Other Words

Isometric exercise is where your muscles flex, but there is no movement. Isotonic exercise takes your muscles through a full range of motion. A full range of motion is best to develop the entire muscle.

The intensity of your upper-body training is important to your progress. Intensity depends on how many reps, sets, how much resistance you use, and how much rest you take between sets.

Duration is how long it takes for you to complete your workout. Your upper-body workout should not take more than an hour. Ideally, each upper-body session should be completed within 45 minutes. Training too long may have a detrimental effect on your adherence.

Frequency is how often you train your upper body, such as two times per week. The rest between workouts allows your upper-body muscles time to recover from the stress of the workout and for them to become toned and stronger.

Evaluate yourself. If your upper-body muscles are feeling stronger and more toned and you're not gaining additional body fat, you are doing everything right.

At first, your body weight is enough resistance. Soon your upper-body muscles will adapt and you may add resistance using bands, free weights, or machine weights. Your goal will be to do your 10 reps with about 75 percent of the maximum resistance you can handle.

When you begin to use resistance, start with a very light weight. Be sure you can perform ten repetitions with perfect form before advancing to a heavier weight. Gradually add weight. Do not increase your resistance more than 5 percent in a single workout.

If you do not have adjustable bands or plates, perform more repetitions at your previous intensity. Most equipment has 10-pound weight increments.

Sets

At first, perform only one set of each exercise. In addition to being time efficient, single-set training is almost as effective as multiple-set training.

Do one exercise each for your chest, back, shoulder, and arm muscles. Always work your larger muscles before your smaller ones. For example, it makes no sense to do a set of close grip push-ups before a set of bench presses. If you fatigue the backs of your arms by doing the close grip push-ups, you won't have enough strength to perform well on the bench press. Both of these exercises target the backs of the arm muscles. The muscles in the backs of your arms become the weak link in the chain.

Instead, do a set of bench presses followed by a set of close grip push-ups. In this case, your chest muscles won't fatigue before the backs of your arms do.

Perform one to three sets per body part.

After you have trained for a few months, your upper-body muscles can handle more than one set of a particular exercise. Do up to three sets of each exercise.

Get It Right

To preserve your shoulder joints, do all exercises in front of the neck instead of behind the neck. For all exercises there is a risk versus benefit. There is no reason to do any exercise pressing from behind the neck because of possible rotator cuff damage and cervical spine injury. And for triceps, the load puts too much stress on a hyper-flexed elbow. There is no need to flex the elbow beyond 90 degrees to train the triceps. A great rule of thumb is that you should always be able to see your hands during any exercise.

If you have a break in form, stop immediately. A break in form signals that you've worked your upper-body muscles enough. Losing your form means you can't finish your reps without changing your body position.

If you're doing a biceps curl and you arch your back, you're finished with the exercise. Whether you've done one set or three sets, once you've groaned out that wobbly rep, you're done. Pay attention to your form rep by rep.

Perform sets consecutively or in a circuit.

If one of your goals is to lose body fat, move quickly from one upper-body exercise to the next. Keep charts to record how you are advancing in each of your muscle groups. Write down how many sets and reps, how much resistance you are using, and how much rest you take between sets. As you increase the resistance and the number of repetitions, your muscles will respond.

When you are ready for an additional challenge, do an upper-body circuit. Perform one set of each exercise without rest. This burns more calories than straight sets of upper-body exercises.

Circuit training also forces your cardiovascular system to work overtime. Without resting between sets, you increase the amount of time you spend toning your upper body compared with the amount of time you spend resting. This increases the metabolic demand of the workout while maintaining your upper-body strength.

Pulsing through your upper-body exercises is another way to add intensity. The principle behind pulsing is that instead of doing full-range-of-motion exercises, you just stay at your mid-range and do partial reps. Pulsing preps your body for using more resistance because it allows you to overload the parts of your upper-body muscles that are strongest, without being limited by the part of the movement where you're weakest.

Do 3 sets of 10 pulsing repetitions, resting one minute between each set. Follow that up with a regular set of 10 full-range-of-motion exercises.

Choose an upper-body exercise that you have difficulty doing a single rep of. Perform 10 sets of 1 repetition, resting 30 seconds between each set.

This is a fabulous workout because you end up performing 10 repetitions of an exercise you normally can only do 1 or 2 reps of. This program requires you to recruit more total muscle fibers than usual.

Reverse your sets and reps. Take your current set and rep scheme and reverse it. Since you normally do 3 sets of 10 reps, try shoulder pressing 10 sets of 3 reps. Since you're stopping at 3 reps instead of 10, rest 10 seconds or less between sets. Reversing your sets and reps allows you to do the same number of total repetitions, but increases the average amount of force your muscles apply during the exercise.

Another way to change your program is to cut your workout in half. Believe it or not, you may be overtraining your upper-body muscles. By reducing the demand on them, you'll allow them to recover. Another option would be to take a week off. When you come back stronger after this break, you'll know you were over-training.

Giant sets consist of performing three different exercises for your upper-body muscles consecutively. Set one is performed, directly followed by a set of the second and third exercise. There is minimal rest between the exercises, but rest between sets is about one minute. For example, do a set of bench presses followed by lat pull-downs, and then shoulder presses.

A superset is performing two different exercises for two opposing muscle groups consecutively. Set one for the fronts of your arms is performed, directly followed by a set for the backs of your arms. There is minimal rest in between the exercises. For example, do a set of reverse curls followed by a set of dips.

Negatives are flexing your upper-body muscles as they lengthen. These are performed by completing a set and then having a training partner help you with the up phase of your exercise. For example, your partner helps you with the up phase of the biceps curl. Then you lower very slowly, unassisted and with total control.

After you have completed a set of 10 repetitions, you should be using enough weight so that your muscles are depleted and cannot perform another rep with perfect form. Your muscles are so fatigued that you need help from your training partner to complete the up phase of any additional reps. Let your partner aid you in the up phase, then you perform the negative portion of the exercise on your own with your partner's guidance.

Reps

Strength gains are not only achieved by increasing the amount of resistance you are using. Increasing the number of repetitions you perform will make your upper body stronger. If you increase the number of repetitions you can perform with good form, you have increased your strength and most likely the muscle tone in your upper-body muscles as well.

But doing hundreds of push-ups in a single workout doesn't adequately challenge your muscles or stimulate your metabolism. First of all, you are probably not performing perfect push-ups, and secondly, if you can do hundreds of push-ups with perfect form, you're overdue for adding resistance.

Do at least 10 repetitions of each exercise.

Doing hundreds of repetitions is kind of like chewing gum. You don't get a trimmed, toned jaw if you chew a lot of gum.

When you train your upper-body muscles, you damage your muscle fibers. After your workout, your body begins to repair those fibers, a process that requires calories.

Added resistance to your upper-body training requires you to use more muscle fibers. You'll increase the number of fibers that are damaged and burn more calories.

Do fewer reps for strength.

Do 10 repetitions for each exercise. Increase the weight and do fewer reps (6 to 8) if your goal is to gain strength in your upper-body muscles. Add enough weight to challenge your upper body but not enough to compromise your form.

Do more reps for endurance

Complete 10 to 12 repetitions with 75 percent of your maximum resistance if your goal is muscular endurance. Ten reps is a good compromise for both absolute strength and muscular endurance.

Rest

Training your upper body two days a week is more than enough. Figure out which days will work best in your busy schedule. Spread your days out to get enough rest between your workouts. Tuesday and Friday works great.

Depending on how many days a week you want to work out, you may split up your routine in a variety of ways. Here is a six-day split routine. You could do chest and triceps on Monday. Back, biceps, and shoulders on Tuesday. And if you have our *Pocket Idiot's Guides to Great Buns and Thighs* and *Great Abs*, you could do legs and abs on Wednesday. Then on Thursday follow your Monday routine, on Friday follow your Tuesday routine, and on Saturday follow your Wednesday routine. You may also do as you please. There are certainly no absolutes when it comes to splitting up your routine. If you are making progress, stick with your program. If you plateau, change things up to shock your muscles.

Your Personal Trainer _____

There are no good or bad exercises. Some are better than others. Choose those that tone your upper body without creating aches and pains.

Rest no longer than a minute between sets.

Rest no longer than a minute between sets of any exercise. Do not dawdle between exercises. If you rest too long you may lose "the pump" and decide to call it a day. Rest a minute between sets of your upper-body workouts. Short, frequent rest periods during a workout are important so that your upper body doesn't burn out too early in your program.

During your rest period, blood delivers oxygen and energy to your upper-body muscles and carries away waste products.

Rest longer on heavy sets and shorter on light sets.

Keep track of how much time you rest between sets in your upper-body workout. As your conditioning improves, perform the same total number of sets and reps, but lessen your rest periods to a maximum of 45 seconds. This requires your muscles to re-cover faster between sets and increases your results.

The harder the set, the more rest you need. One way to maximize your time is to superset upper-body exercises, and take less rest between sets. Do a set of flyes for the chest followed immediately by a set of seated rowing for the back.

Take at least two days rest between workouts.

Your upper-body muscles should be given 48-72 hours of rest before attacking them again. Your muscles firm up between training days. However, too much rest between workouts can hurt your progress. In as little as 96 hours, the benefits of your hard upper-body work can begin to disappear.

Chapter 4

Tone at Home

In This Chapter

- Convenient and efficient at any level
- Get long, lean muscles
- Quick workouts, fast results
- New muscle appearing everywhere
- Sexy arms and shoulders

There's no place like home for training convenience. You don't have to drive anywhere, the weather is never a problem, and you don't have to worry about parking. Best of all, you can exercise in your pajamas and no one will care. At home, you don't have to talk to anyone. If you feel uncomfortable around hard bodies, you won't have to see them, either. And you may not enjoy working out around people of the opposite sex. You don't have to wait for machines or hear the endless clanging of weights, and you don't have to wipe sweat off machines. At home there are fewer distractions than in the gym. Most important, you won't have a monthly gym payment.

No gym equipment is necessary to develop firm arms, a tapered back, and a well-defined chest. On all tone-at-home upper-body exercises, keep your back straight, stomach in, neck relaxed, and head up. Perform each exercise 3 seconds up and 3 seconds down through a full range of motion. Perform 10 repetitions of each exercise exhaling on the exertion phase of each rep. Focus on the muscles you are training and relax the others. If an exercise is too difficult, choose another one.

Modified Push-Ups

Modified Push-Ups are the best exercise for your upper body. You firm your chest, back, arms, and shoulders. The rest of your body has to support your movement, too.

Keep your back straight and knees slightly bent so that a straight line could be drawn from the back of your head to the back of your heels. At first, don't concern yourself with how far you descend. The up position is a workout in itself. As you get stronger, go down further until eventually your elbows bend at 90 degrees.

Do not rest in the up or the down position. Do not fully extend your elbows in the up position. Your elbows should always remain soft (slightly bent). Move slowly through each repetition so that you could stop at any point during the rep and maintain perfect form.

Be careful that your back doesn't sag as you fatigue. Lead with your chest and resist the temptation to drop your head. Your head should always stay in line with your spine. Begin doing modified push-ups on the wall. When you can do 10 repetitions with perfect form, do them from the floor on your knees. When you can do 10 reps with perfect form, try them from your feet. You can also use a stability ball to make the exercise easier or more difficult.

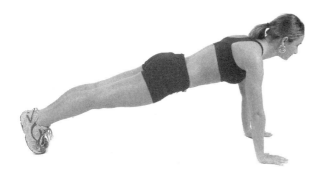

1. Your hands are shoulder-width apart on the wall or on the floor. If you are on the floor, you may begin on your knees or on your feet.

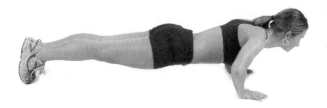

2. Lower your chest a few inches by bending your elbows 90 degrees.

3. Return to your starting position by extending your elbows.

In Other Words

Your pectoralis major and pectoralis minor muscles are the muscles of your chest. They may be toned and tightened from several different angles.

Close Grip Push-Ups

Close Grip Push-Ups zone in on the backs of your arms and the fronts of your shoulders. This is one of the best exercises for the backs of your arms.

The back of your body should be a perfectly slanted ramp from the top of your head to the back of your heel. Don't allow your head to drop or move to either side. Your head should always stay in line with your spine.

Lead with your chest on each repetition. Keep your
upper arms near your sides. Do not allow your elbows
to flare out or lock in the up-position. If your wrists
or elbows hurt when you perform this exercise,
spread your hands out until you are pain-free. Do
not rest in the up or the down position. Keep your
elbows in close to your body and your back straight
throughout the duration of the exercise.

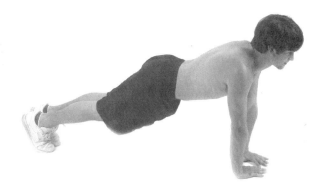

1. Your hands are together creating a diamond
   shape with your fingers on the wall or on
   the floor. If you are on the floor, you may
   begin on your knees or on your feet.

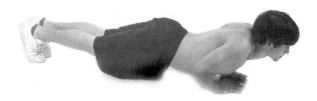

2. Lower your chest a few inches by bending
   your elbows to a 90 degree angle, keeping
   the elbows close to the body.

3. Return to your starting position by extending your elbows.

Bet You Didn't Know

Any movement where you flex your
elbows in a pulling motion tones the
fronts of your arms. Any movement that
extends your elbows tones the backs of
your arms.

Dips

Dips tighten the backs of your arms, chest, and
shoulders. Don't round your back or bend your
elbows too much. Keep your back straight, elbows
in, shoulders down, and chest out.

Begin each exercise by drawing your navel into
your spine. At first, bend your arms only slightly
for each rep. As you get stronger, bend your arms
further until you max out at 90 degrees. Never

bend your elbows further than 90 degrees. In the up position, keep your elbows soft.

If this exercise is too difficult, allow your legs to boost you back into the up position on each rep. An advanced form of this exercise would be to place a weight in your lap when you perform your repetitions.

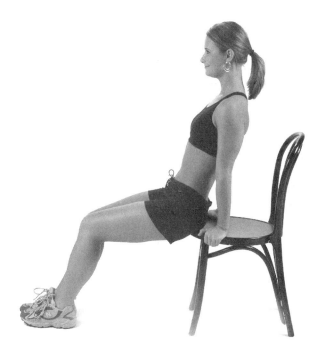

1. Sit on the edge of a chair with your hands behind you and your palms facing downward.

2. Keep your hands shoulder-width apart and extend your legs out to the front.

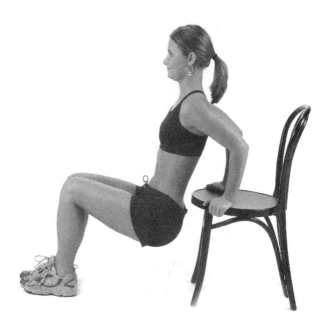

3. Brace yourself with your hands as you lower yourself a few inches by bending your elbows.

4. Return to your original position by extending your elbows.

Your Personal Trainer

If you have a twinge of discomfort as you move through any exercise, find a different range of motion to prevent pain and possible injury.

Chest Fly on Floor

The Chest Fly on the Floor shapes up your chest. Begin each exercise by drawing your navel into your spine. Flex your chest muscles as you move through your range of motion. Imagine flexing your chest muscles together so that a nickel wouldn't fall out from between them.

Concentrate on flexing your chest on both the upward and the downward motion to get maximum results. Keep your elbows bent at all times and be sure that both arms move together. Shoulders should stay down and your head should rest on the floor. When you can perform 10 repetitions with perfect form, add more weight.

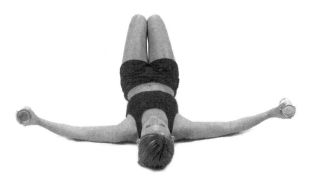

1. Lie on your back with your arms out to the side with your elbows slightly bent. Hold a light can in each hand.

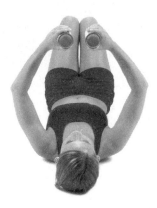

2. Bring your arms together toward the middle of your chest as if you were hugging a tree— not too straight or bent, just a slight curve at the elbow.

3. Return to your original position, bringing your arms in the same path that you did when you brought them together.

Single Arm Rowing with Chair

The Single Arm Rowing with Chair gives your back that hourglass shape. Begin in a position of stability. Draw your navel into your spine. Keep your upper body square to the floor for the duration of the exercise. Resist the temptation to twist your upper body.

The first movement you make should be your shoulder blade moving toward the ceiling. It is particularly important on this exercise not to jerk the weight up. Be sure to keep your back tabletop flat and don't bring your elbow up too high.

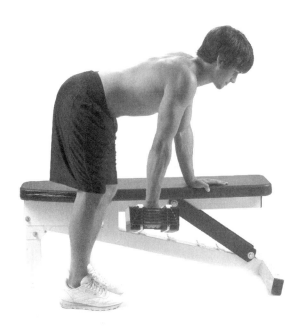

1. Stand next to a chair and bend from your hips with your left hand supporting your body on the chair and your right arm extended by your side. Keep your back straight during the entire exercise. Hold onto a can with your right hand.

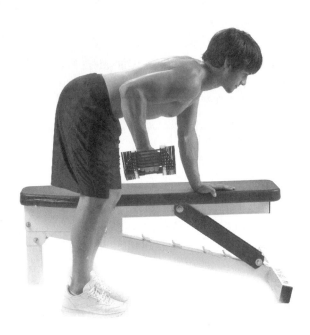

2. Pull the can up to your side by lifting your elbow toward the ceiling.

3. Return to the starting position moving your arm along the same path.

Get It Right

Be careful not to fully extend your elbows or knees on any exercise as that takes the resistance off your muscles and puts pressure on your joints.

Lateral Arm Raise

The Lateral Arm Raise builds the sides of your shoulders. You may never have to wear shoulder pads again. Perform this exercise seated or standing.

Begin by drawing your navel into your spine. Keep your back straight and move slowly so that you are not throwing the weights. You should be able to stop at any point during the lift and maintain perfect form. Keep your elbows slightly bent throughout the movement and bring your hands no higher than shoulder level.

If this exercise is too difficult, lighten the weight or bend your elbows 90 degrees. To make this exercise more challenging, extend your elbows until they are just slightly bent. For further isolation, you may perform all of your repetitions with one arm and then repeat with your other arm.

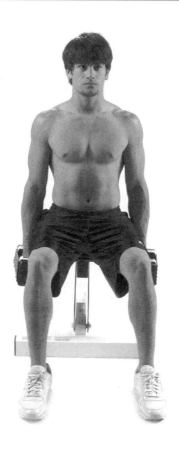

1. Begin by sitting with your feet shoulder-width apart and your arms held to your sides with your elbows slightly bent.

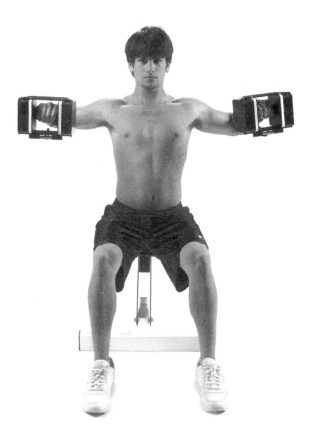

2. Keep your elbows bent as you raise both arms up from your sides until they are parallel to the floor.

3. Return to your original position, keeping your arms moving in the same path.

Chapter 5

Muscle Makeover

In This Chapter

- Work out at work
- Real results in a short time
- Use your desk to train your chest
- Get toned while you're on the phone

Upper body training in your office is fun because there are so many different exercises to choose from. Close your office door so nobody sees you working out on company time. Do a set of 10 repetitions and then write that important memo. During your next set, ponder a company takeover. The great thing is that you won't sweat bullets because you are cooling down between sets, writing memos, and answering the phone. Your creativity will improve when you add mini-workouts to your day. Your colleagues will marvel at your always-pumped, well-defined arms.

Treat your office workouts just as you would your gym workouts. Your chest muscles don't care whether they are pressing a bar or a desk. Train each upper-body muscle group no more than twice a week, but if you enjoy working out daily, split up your body parts. On Monday, train your chest and the backs of your arms. On Tuesday, work your back, shoulders, and the fronts of your arms. You could even tone a single muscle group each day.

Use perfect posture on every exercise. Hold your head up, shoulders back, stomach in, and chest out. Perform 10 repetitions of each exercise. Be careful not to lock your elbows. Begin each movement by drawing your navel in toward your spine using your lower abdominal muscles. Continue to flex those muscles through the duration of your reps. Breathe normally or exhale on the exertion of each rep.

In Other Words

Your triceps consist of three muscles in the back of your arm. These muscles are used to extend your elbow for pushing movements.

Push-Ups Off Your Desk

Push-Ups Off Your Desk are great for your chest, the backs of your arms, and shoulders. Make sure your desk is secured to the floor!

Performing desk push-ups is less challenging than doing them from the floor, so you may have to do several sets in order to fatigue your muscles. Draw an imaginary line from the top of your head to the back of your heel. Keep your wrist neutral and don't allow your back to sag.

Move slowly through each repetition—three seconds down, three seconds up. If it is too difficult to do a regular desk push-up, just bend your elbows a couple of inches on each rep. As you get stronger, increase your range of motion. Never go beyond a 90-degree angle with your elbows. After a few months, you can challenge yourself further by stopping for three seconds every inch on your repetition down and every inch on your repetition up.

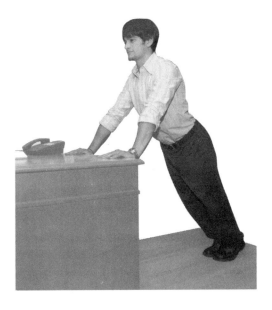

1. Stand about a foot away from your desk and place your hands shoulder-width apart on the top edge of your desk.

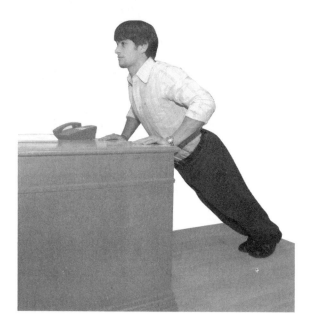

2. Lead with your chest as you lower your body toward the desk by bending your elbows.

3. When your elbows bend to 90 degrees, press back into your original position.

Your Personal Trainer _____

Don't baby yourself during your office
workouts. Your muscles don't know
whether stimulation comes from a
weight machine or pressing against the
back of your chair.

Dips

Dips tighten the backs of your arms, shoulders, and
chest. Make sure that your desk is secured to the
floor. Sit on the edge of your desk or chair and (as
soon as no one's watching) begin your repetitions.

Maintain perfect posture throughout the duration
of the exercise. At first, bend your elbows an inch
or two on each repetition. You may rest in the up
position if you need to. Use your legs to help you
move up and down.

As you become stronger, bend your elbows a little
more. Be careful not to bend your elbows further
than 90 degrees. Move slowly through each repetition. Breathe normally or exhale on the exertion
phase of each rep. As you become more advanced,
do not rest in the up or the down position and do
not use your legs to help complete your reps.

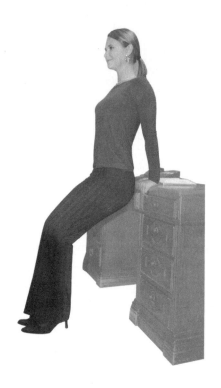

1. Stand with your back to your desk and your hands placed behind you on your desk with your fingers pointed forward.

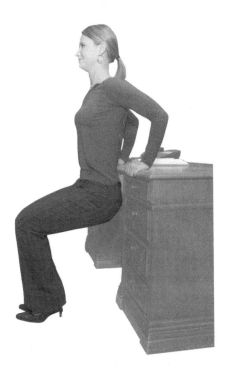

2. Use your legs for balance as you lower yourself by bending your elbows.

3. Extend your elbows and return to your starting position.

Squeeze the Desk

Squeeze the Desk firms the muscles in your chest. At first do not squeeze hard. Press with the palms and heels of your hands. Focus on your chest muscles flexing. As you get stronger, you may press harder.

Be sure to breathe normally while you are doing this exercise. Do not hold your breath. If you prefer, you may exhale through each repetition. If holding each repetition for three seconds is too challenging, begin with one second. Add a second a week until you can hold your desk press for three seconds.

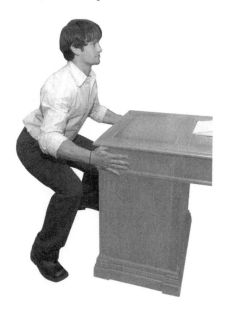

1. Face the narrow part of your desk. Place both palms on the outside of your desk with your elbows bent.

2. Press your palms into the desk, flexing your chest muscles. Hold for three seconds. Then relax.

3. Be sure to keep your back straight whether you squat down by bending your knees or lean over hinging at your hips.

 Bet You Didn't Know _____

> Pushing and pulling exercises are all you need to firm and tone your upper body.

Shoulder Flexion

Shoulder Flexion firms and tones the fronts of your shoulders. Perform this exercise either sitting or standing. Try this move from different angles so that you will firm and tone all parts of the fronts of your shoulders. For example, moving from a seated to a standing position changes the angle of the exercise.

If you are performing the exercise with your left arm, place your right hand on your left shoulder and feel the muscle flex. Be sure to breathe normally through the entire movement. If you prefer, you may exhale through each rep.

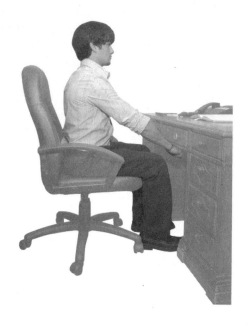

1. Sit in a military posture with the back of your right hand contacting the underside of your desk. (Keep your chest out, stomach in, shoulders back, and your head up.) Keep your elbow slightly bent.

2. Flex the front of your shoulder, pressing the back of your hand into the desk as if you are trying to lift it. Hold for three seconds. Then relax.

Back Exercise

Back Exercise adds form to your upper back. Before you begin this exercise, try it without moving. Simply grab the bottom of your chair with both hands, keep your back straight, and pull gently. You should feel the muscles in your back flex. These are the muscles you will be using to perform this exercise.

Be sure to breathe normally through the duration or, if you prefer, you may exhale through each rep. Use your arms as if they were hooks so that they do not fatigue. On the way up you are training your back. On the way down, you are training both your abs and your back. Keep your neck relaxed throughout.

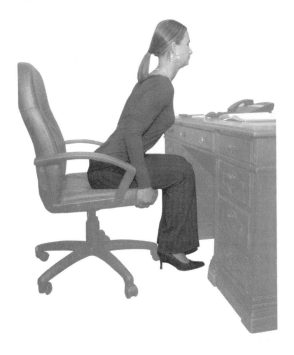

1. Grab the underside of your chair with your hands. While seated in your chair, pull your stomach in, and bend forward with your back straight, hinging from your hips.

2. Hold onto the underside of your chair as you extend your back to your original position.

Get It Right

Be sure you maintain a balance between the musculature of the fronts of your arms and the backs of your arms to promote symmetry and prevent injury.

Doorknob Pull-Ups

Doorknob Pull-Ups firm your arms and back. This is a great full-body exercise because all of your muscles take part in the movement. Even your forearms get a great workout from gripping the doorknob.

As the muscles in your arms and back begin to fatigue, allow your legs to help you through each rep. As a further challenge, after you have completed your 10 reps, allow your legs to push you up into the start position, but on the way down use your arms and back to slow your descent. Be sure to use your legs for balance.

(Don't let your colleagues catch you doing this exercise or it will be very difficult to explain!)

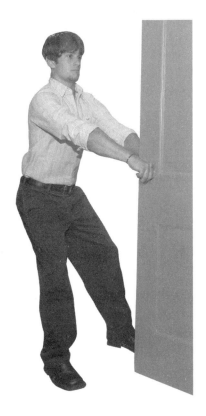

1. Grab one doorknob in each hand.

2. Using your legs for balance, sink toward the floor as your arms extend.

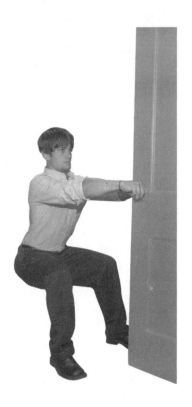

3. Pull yourself back up. Use your legs if necessary.

Chapter 6

Cut and Defined

In This Chapter

- Fixing those problem areas
- Trim your arms
- Enjoy the burn
- It won't work if you don't do it
- Better workout, shorter time

The gym is a virtual paradise if you want to cut and define your upper body. With so many exercises and machines to choose from, you almost can't go wrong. But you *can* go wrong if you train too hard, too much, or with improper form.

Maintain perfect posture on all of your upper-body exercises. When in doubt, assume the military "attention" position. Keep your elbows slightly bent on all exercises. Never bring a bar behind your neck. Move slowly through each exercise so that you could stop at any given moment if necessary. Focus on the muscle group you're training and allow all your other muscles to relax. Be sure the amount of weight that you use doesn't hurt your form.

If you begin to lose your form, stop the exercise immediately. If your muscles are sore from a previous workout, train a different body part. Move through a full range of motion on each exercise. Begin each exercise by using your lower abdominals to draw your navel into your spine. Exhale during the exertion phase of each rep.

> ### Bet You Didn't Know
>
> Performing just one set of an exercise gives you 80 percent of the benefits of doing three sets.

Bench Press

The Bench Press focuses on your chest and the backs of your arms—it's the king of all upper-body exercises. Although gym rats may ask you how much you can bench, a more important question might be, "How do your chest and the backs of your arms look?"

Keep your thumbs under the bar and press your hands toward each other to keep your chest muscles flexed throughout the lift. When you lower the bar toward your chest, pause when your elbows are parallel to the floor and then exhale as you press the bar up. The bar will find its own path to the top of the range of motion, and it is generally not straight up and down. Your body naturally finds angles where your body is stronger. You can lift heavier weight with free weights where you can alter the angle of

your lift. When you try to lift the same amount of
weight on a machine that does not allow you to vary
the angle of your lift, it will feel 10 pounds heavier.

After you press the weight up to the top, squeeze
your chest muscles together as if you were trying to
hold a nickel between them. Flex the backs of your
arms, too.

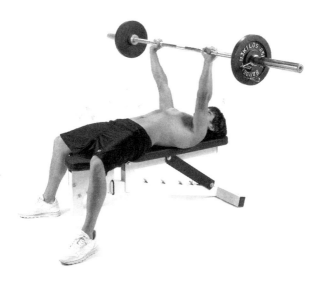

1. Lie down with your back on the bench and
   your hands holding the weights shoulder-
   width apart. Squeeze your shoulder blades
   together in preparation for your lift.

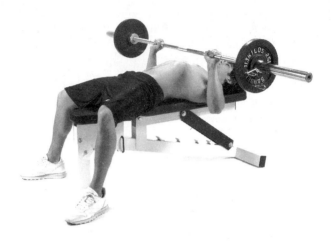

2. Bend your elbows as you control the weight, slowly inching down until your elbows are parallel to the floor.

3. Slowly extend your elbows, returning to your starting position.

Triceps Press

The Triceps Press firms the backs of your arms. In fact, any exercise where you extend your elbows trains your triceps, so if this exercise doesn't meet your needs, find another angle where you are extending your elbows.

The main part of this exercise that tones your triceps is the last few inches just before you reach full extension on the up phase. Do not fully lock your elbows, but move to a position as close to lockout as possible. The only joints that should be moving are your elbows, to isolate the triceps and prevent other muscles from helping. Do not bend your elbows past 90 degrees on the down phase.

Get It Right

To protect your shoulders on the bench press, lighten the weight and never let your elbows drop lower than parallel to the floor.

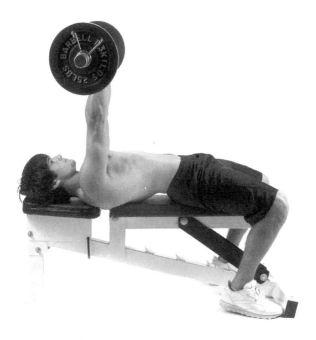

1. Lie down on your back and hold the weights above your chest with your elbows almost fully extended.

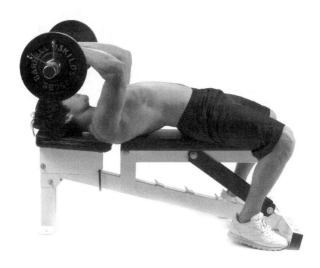

2. Lower the weights toward your forehead very slowly until your elbows bend at 90 degrees.

3. Extend your elbows back to your starting position.

Lat Pull-Down

The Lat Pull-Down widens your upper back to create that "V" shape. Lead with your elbows and keep your body still. You may use either an overhand or underhand grip.

The first movement you make should be to squeeze your shoulder blades together and press them down. Instead of jerking the bar, just by squeezing and depressing your shoulder blades you have stimulated activity in your lat muscles.

Resist the tendency to pull with your arms.
Imagine your hands are hooks on the bar so that
you do not squeeze too tightly.

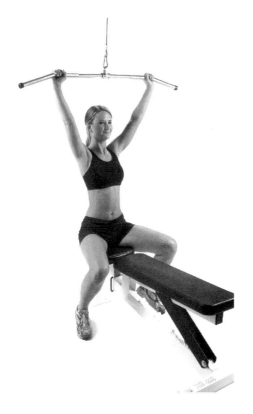

1. Begin seated with your hands shoulder-width
    apart on the lat pull-down bar. Set the position
    of the seat on the machine appropriately to
    avoid compromising your form.

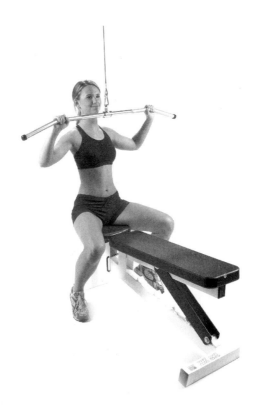

2. Pull the bar down to your upper chest.

Maintain perfect form on the negative portion of this exercise by keeping your chest out and your back straight. Move very slowly and feel a full stretch on your lat muscle at the end of each rep.

In Other Words

Your **latissimus dorsi** is your upper-back muscle. There is no truth to the myth that if you use an extra-wide grip it widens your upper back even more.

Seated Rowing

Seated Rowing firms the muscles of your middle back. These are the muscles between your shoulder blades. This is a very simple exercise, but you will see people in gyms make it very difficult and even dangerous.

The worst mistake you can make on this exercise is to lean forward or lean back. Even though it is called "Seated Rowing" most people tend to perform the exercise by leaning back or "rowing" rather than keeping their back straight. Keep your chest out as you pull the handles toward your chest. Keep your arms close to your sides so that your inner upper arm brushes by the side of your chest. Once again your hands are like hooks, so that you don't use other muscles to jerk the weight forward.

At the completion of the movement, imagine the backs of your elbows as wings so that your elbows move toward each other.

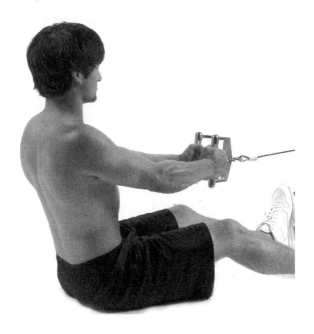

1. Begin in a seated position. Grab a handle with each hand with your elbows almost fully extended and your knees slightly bent.

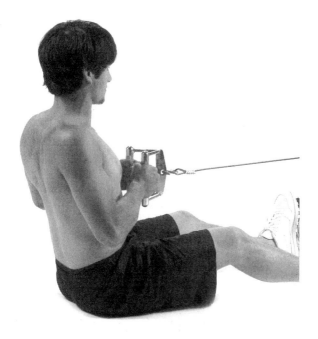

2. Pull the handles toward your chest, keeping your elbows in close to your sides.

Allow the resistance to pull your hands back to the starting position until you feel a full stretch on your lats. Be sure to keep your chest out, stomach in, and back straight for the duration of all of your reps.

Shoulder Press

The Shoulder Press sculpts all three parts of your shoulder. Always press from the front of your neck instead of the back. You may perform this exercise seated or standing, but keep perfect posture throughout.

In the down position, your elbows should bend no further than 90 degrees. In the up position, extend your elbows until if you pressed up any further they would lock. Pause at the top. Flex the backs of your arms and lift your shoulders as if you were trying to touch your ears.

It doesn't matter whether you use barbells or dumbbells for this exercise. It is also your choice (if you use dumbbells instead of a straight bar) to either twist the elbows up into position or keep your palms facing forward.

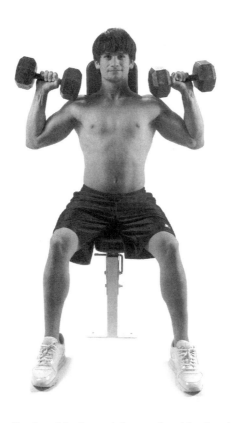

1. Begin with the weights at shoulder level.

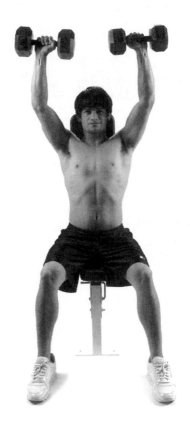

2. Extend your elbows over your head until they are almost straight.

3. Return your arms back to the starting position.

Your Personal Trainer _____

Strong muscles take over for weak or injured ones. Do not neglect your weaker muscles. If you don't use them, you'll lose them.

Biceps Curl

The Biceps Curl works the front of your upper arm. You may use a barbell or dumbbells for this exercise. Keep your body still during the entire exercise.

If you use dumbbells, you can perform this exercise either seated or standing. With a barbell you must stand throughout the exercise.

Move very slowly, because many people accidentally cheat on this exercise by bending the back and "kipping" the weight up. Another common mistake people make is to not go through the full range of motion, and cheat with half-reps. At the bottom of the rep, flex your triceps for a split second. Let your biceps do the work and you will see great results. Move slowly through both the up and the down phases, keeping constant tension on your biceps.

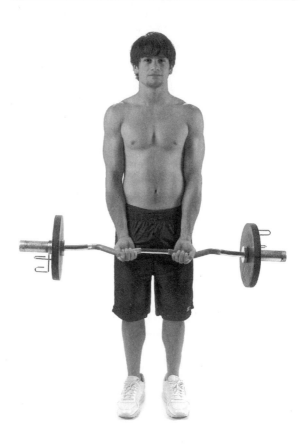

1. Begin in a standing position with your palms facing forward and the weights near your thighs with your elbows slightly bent.

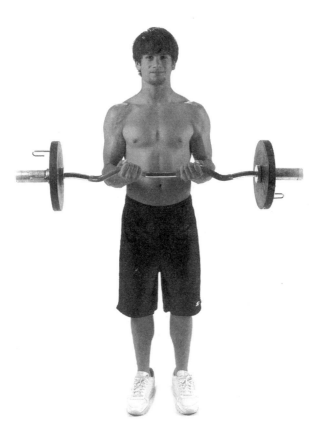

2. Bend your elbows up slowly to a 45 degree angle.

3. Return to your starting position with the weights traveling the same path as on the upward pull.

Reverse Curl

The Reverse Curl tones your forearms and the fronts of your upper arms. Press your feet firmly into the floor and resist the temptation to lean back, lift up on your toes, or move your feet. Keep your wrists in line with your forearms. Keep your elbows close to your body.

Be sure you use a light weight for this exercise. You may use an E-Z Curl bar, dumbbells, or a straight bar to complete this movement.

Maintain perfect posture throughout the exercise with the elbows as the only moveable joint. Resist the temptation to swing the weight up into position. Keep your knees bent and back straight throughout.

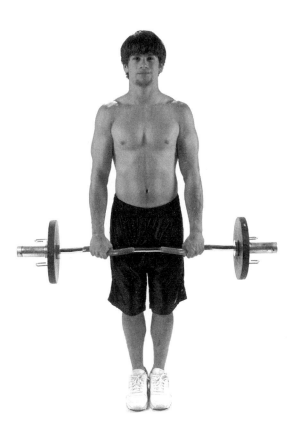

1. Begin in a standing position with your palms facing backward and the weights near your thighs with your elbows slightly bent.

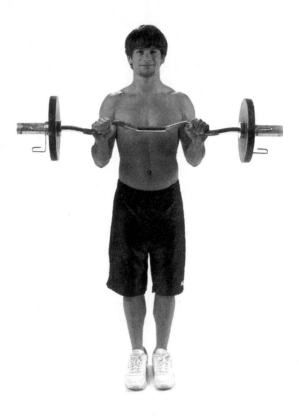

2. Bend your elbows up slowly to a 45 degree angle.

3. Return to your starting position with the weights traveling the same path.

Chapter 7

Lean Body

In This Chapter

- You are a fat-burning machine
- Sculpt a slimmer upper body
- Fewer exercises—quality workout
- Tone on your own
- Stretch and shape

This chapter summarizes an overall philosophy, combining different programs to achieve a defined, balanced, and riveting upper body in a healthy way. Use a combination of strength, cardiovascular, and flexibility training. Each section provides you with the basics to get you started on the program today. Learn how you can train indoors, outdoors, or while watching TV.

There are powerful forces that try to drag you back to the couch. You will learn to make your upper-body routine fit into your busy life. You should never spend more than 10 minutes training each muscle group. If you work a body part more than 10 minutes, you're overtraining. Not only does this promise diminishing returns, it sets you up for overuse injuries.

The mode of training you choose should vary according to your time, energy level, and goals. Attack your upper-body muscles at different angles. This helps you to recruit more muscle fibers to enhance your training effect.

Your upper-body muscles adapt to your workout, so you must occasionally "shock" them to enhance your progress. Change your workout periodically to get an upper body you can be proud of.

Your Favorite Sitcom Is Your Workout

Work out while you watch your favorite TV show. In a two-hour program there are 30 minutes of commercials. During each commercial, get off of the couch and move!

Push-ups are the greatest upper-body workout you can do during commercials. Begin in a push-up position on your hands and feet. Complete as many push-ups as possible.

As your arms and shoulders fatigue, drop to your knees until you cannot do another push-up. By then the commercial is over and you get to take a long break until your next set of push-ups.

Bet You Didn't Know

> A toned upper body means that your muscles are firing constantly. Keep those muscles firing by training consistently.

The faster you move, the faster you will see definition and separation in your upper-body muscles. But start slowly and progress gradually. If you jump up and down as high as you can for a two-minute commercial you won't be able to get off the couch for your next bout of exercise. Walk, march, jog, and run, and eventually you might decide to jump.

Indoor Training

The best bet for toning and defining your upper body without becoming fanatical is to combine pushing and pulling. All of the muscles in your chest, back, shoulders, and arms, can be trained with variations of two exercises—pull-ups and push-ups.

To get a cardio workout and strengthen and tone every muscle in your upper body in a minimum amount of time, superset push-ups and pull-ups. Perform each set to failure. Failure simply means when you experience a break in your form.

- Cycle I is a set of wide grip pull-ups with an overhand grip. Then do a set of wide grip push-ups. Take a 30-second break.

- Cycle II is a set of close grip pull-ups with an underhand grip. Then do a set of close grip push-ups. Take a 30-second break.
- Cycle III is a set of shoulder-width grip pull-ups with an underhand grip. Then do a set of shoulder-width push-ups with your feet spread.

Don't be discouraged if you cannot do one push-up or pull-up. Moving quickly between sets and cycles keeps your heart rate up. Some people prefer pounding the pavement, but they don't get the muscular endurance and upper-body toning.

In Other Words

You lose adipose tissue (fat) over your whole body over time. That is, you cannot lose fat on the back of your arm just by working your triceps.

Mix and match your exercise options and you will never get bored—but it's not just mental. If you do the same exercises day in and day out, you will get the same results. Soon, your muscles adapt and there will be no improvement.

Your upper body needs to be challenged or your muscles stagnate. Cross-training keeps you in great shape. Find a rock-climbing wall for Day One of your workout. Day Two you can swim. Day Three is cross-country skiing. And Day Four is an indoor elliptical machine with the upper-body option.

Your Personal Trainer _____

Stretch after your workout, not between sets of upper-body exercises. Stretching between sets makes you weaker for your next set.

Outdoor Training

If you have a yard, you don't need to spend hours in the gym training your abs. Use a push mower, and Lawn Mowing Day is an upper-body workout!

You can also get a great workout raking, gardening, and shoveling snow. You will be amazed at the intensity of your workout. Pushing, pulling, dragging, and cornering challenge your chest, back, shoulders, and arms at different angles better than the best celebrity-infomercial gizmo.

Stretching Your Upper Body

Many of the strengthening exercises that you do for your upper body stretch your muscles at the end of your range of motion. For example, when you extend your elbows for your biceps curl, you stretch the fronts of your arms. The lat pull-down or pull-up stretch your back and chest.

However, it's a good idea for you to set aside a few minutes after each workout for stretching.

Get It Right _____

Hold your stretch instead of bouncing. Bouncing through your stretches may cause micro-tears in your muscles, damaging the fibers.

In fact, it's best to stretch at the completion of your workout to help prevent cramps and soreness. Warm up before you stretch. If you can find a warm room, that helps your muscles to relax and elongate. Relax into each stretch and concentrate on lengthening the belly of the muscle. Exhale as you move into each position. Learn to hold your stretch at least 10 seconds in order to fully relax the muscle. Add 2 seconds a week until you work up to 30 seconds. Within months you may stretch to a slight level of tension, but never approaching pain.

Triceps Stretch

The Triceps Stretch lengthens the back of your upper arm. Keep your back straight, shoulders down, and neck aligned with your back. Resist the temptation to drop your head forward. Flexible triceps are important for any throwing motion. Be careful not to bring your elbow back too far behind your head.

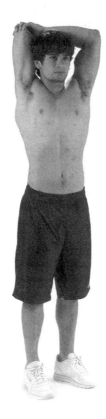

1. Stand with your feet shoulder-width apart
    and your knees slightly bent. Reach back
    with your right arm as if you were trying to
    scratch the middle of your back. Your right
    elbow is now beside your ear. Grab your
    elbow with your left hand.

2. Pull your elbow gently toward the ceiling
    until you feel a stretch.

3. Switch arms and repeat.

Shoulder Stretch

The Shoulder Stretch loosens up the muscles in your shoulder. Maintaining shoulder flexibility is important for just about every upper-body movement that you make.

Keep your shoulders parallel to the floor, your back straight, and your eyes looking over the horizon. Resist the temptation to twist your entire upper body.

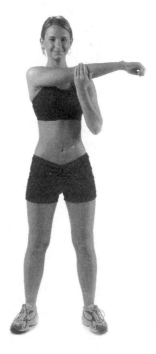

1. Stand with your feet shoulder-width apart and your knees slightly bent. Bring your right arm across your body so that your right elbow is in front of your chest.

2. Grab the back of your right upper arm with your left hand and gently pull to the left.

3. Switch arms and repeat.

Chest Stretch

The Chest Stretch lengthens the muscles in your upper, middle, and lower chest. Flexibility in your chest will maintain your posture. If your chest is tight, your shoulders roll forward into a slumping pattern.

Keep your shoulders parallel and down throughout this stretching exercise. Keep your chin up and your chest out.

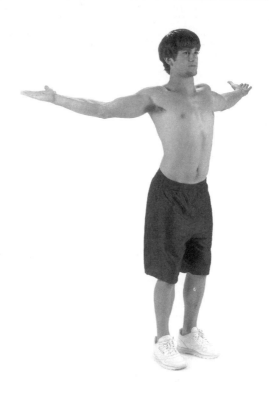

1. Stand with your feet shoulder-width apart and your knees slightly bent. Extend your arms out to the side with your palms facing up.

2. Flex the muscles in your middle back to pull your arms back. Hold when you feel the stretch in your chest.

Upper-Back Stretch

The Upper-Back Stretch lengthens the muscles in the upper part of your back. This is a "feel good" stretch. Bring your chin down to your chest and relax into the stretch. If you suffer from knee problems, do this exercise standing, while facing a wall.

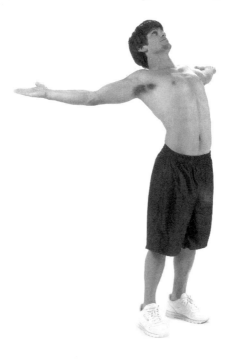

1. Move to the floor on your hands and knees. Bend your knees into a fully flexed position.

2. Keep your hands where they are so that when you bend your knees you feel a stretch in your upper back.

Chapter **8**

Feed Your Muscle

In This Chapter

- Slimming secrets are easy
- Bulge be gone; losing back fat
- Eating to lose
- Eat a lot, lose a lot
- Feed your muscle, starve the fat

To slim down the flab on the backs of your arms, you have to eat right. The subcutaneous fat between your skin and muscle is the problem. This eating program is the solution.

Short-term diets lead to short-term results. If you stop eating carbs, you lose weight, but you gain it back. The scale doesn't tell you that you only lost water and muscle. When your weight returns, you can't see your well-shaped arms under the fluff.

How Diets Work

You tried low-carb diets but your cravings were so powerful that you finally gave in. Even before low-carb diets, liquid low-calorie fasts were popular.

But here's the thing: when you do not eat enough, your body naturally slows its energy expenditure. Whether it is a famine or just a long time between feedings, your body has a protective mechanism so you do not need to eat as much food during lean times. That worked great during caveman days. Unfortunately, in times of plenty, nature's protective energy conservation translates into a coating of fat surrounding your never-to-be-noticed upper body.

Bet You Didn't Know

> You lose weight quickly on a low-carb diet, but what the scale doesn't tell you is most of your weight loss is water and muscle.

The Carbs that Count

Carbs aren't good for you—*they're fantastic!* The controversy is that there are different kinds of carbs. Processed carbs are man-made, refined, and contain a lot of calories per serving. Close-to-the-ground carbs are nutrient-dense. They are packed with vitamins, minerals, and fiber. Most fruits and veggies contain fewer calories than processed carbs.

These nutrient-dense carbs give you the energy you need without adding fat to your well-defined physique. There has never been a single case of someone getting fat by eating apples and oranges.

Colorful veggies such as sweet potatoes, tomatoes, kale, spinach, broccoli, peppers, and carrots are vitamin arsenals that you cannot get enough of. The deeper and darker the color, the better for your body. So eat as many and as often as possible.

Fruits and veggies and whole grains provide you with quick energy to power your upper-body workouts. They also contain fiber and other compounds that are essential to uncovering those rippling triceps. Nutrient-dense carbs are your muscles' best source of energy—they're rocket fuel for your chest and back muscles. Feed your muscle and starve your fat. Eat and drink just enough to satisfy.

Calorically dense processed, refined, and man-made carbs such as white flour, bagels, pasta, and boxed cereals are packed with calories you probably don't need. If you're a marathon runner or ultra-distance cyclist, you burn up these extra calories. But if you work a desk job and don't have the luxury of being able to run, bike, or swim several hours a day, eat nutrient-dense carbs instead.

The bottom line? Carbs aren't the problem, too many calories are. Don't eat more calories than you use and your arms won't turn to mush.

Protein for Power

Besides nutrient-dense carbs, another major staple in your diet is lean protein. Eat a serving of protein at each meal. (A "serving" of anything will be about the size of a deck of cards.)

Protein slow-releases carbs so that you feel full longer. This nourishes your muscles and decreases fat stores surrounding the hard-earned muscles of your upper body. Protein is also the foundation for your muscle. Besides water and nutrient-dense carbs, protein is the most important macro-nutrient in your upper-body–sculpting program.

Lean proteins include sirloin tip, eye of round, and round steak. Small chickens are leaner than larger ones, and turkey breast is leaner than chicken. Pork tenderloin and Canadian bacon are the leanest pork cuts. If you are a vegetarian, eat protein-rich low-fat dairy and lots of beans and legumes. Kidney beans, dried peas, lentils, and other types of beans are good sources of protein. Peas and beans are digested slowly for a steady release of energy. For people on the go, supplementing protein shakes is easy with whey protein and the pre-packaged shakes that are available. They are easy, convenient, and simple to do!

Fat Can Be Your Friend

Carbs and protein have four calories per gram. That doesn't mean much until you find out that fat has nine calories per gram. Combine a serving of protein and a serving of carbs and it doesn't equal one serving of fat.

Fat has more than twice the calories as protein or carbs, but fat is not your enemy. You just need to eat the right kind of fat.

Drizzle a tablespoon of olive oil, flaxseed oil, or canola oil into your eating program. Eat omega-three fatty acids, which are found in fish, whenever you can.

Fat is important in your diet because it makes you feel full. You may eat all of the carbs in the house, but until you eat a morsel containing some fat, you may not be satisfied.

Fat disperses flavors across your tongue. This gives your taste buds a chance to allow you to experience a wide range of flavors (sweet, sour, spicy) to create a feeling of satiety or satisfaction.

Omega-three fatty acids from fish, flaxseed oil, and canola oil improve nerve conduction, lubricate your joints and skin, and have been touted as the next miracle anti-aging agent.

 Your Personal Trainer

Grab a handful of seeds or nuts. Peanut butter on whole wheat is also a great source of essential fat.

The Universal Solvent

Add some water to the recipe and you've got yourself a program. You need water as a coolant, to digest and absorb food, transport nutrients, build and rebuild cells, remove waste products, and enhance circulation.

Most people walk around dehydrated. Drink about 64 ounces of water a day. But if you work out hard, drink more than that. If it's dry and hot, or if you are sweating profusely, drink liberally. Water by itself won't chisel those abs, but it keeps your metabolism revved.

Eat to Fuel Your Muscles

What you learned in health class is still true: *a balanced diet of fruits and veggies works.* Add a portion of lean protein with a tablespoon of your favorite healthy essential fat and you're on your way to that lean upper body you deserve!

After eating correctly becomes a habit, you will look forward to feeding your chest, back, shoulder, and arm muscles quality food every few hours. Eat right most of the time and you are on the program. You will have bad eating days and that's okay. Bad days are part of the eating program.

Your body uses smaller meals more efficiently. When you eat a huge meal, the body uses what it needs and stores the rest in your fat cells.

Your Daily Diet

You may want to also consider adjusting your nutritional intake, time, frequency, and so on according to your schedule/activities. Figure out the foods that work for you. You may prefer to eat most of your starchy carbs through the day and cut back on them in the evening. Eat breakfast like a king, lunch like a queen, and dinner like a pauper.

If you want to keep your upper body toned and strong, *eat breakfast!* After fasting all night, your muscles need energy. Eating breakfast not only increases your energy, but you will make better food choices for the rest of the day. A good breakfast is oatmeal or a low-sugar cold cereal, non-fat milk, and a banana or raisins.

Eat a lean roast beef sandwich for lunch. Between lunch and dinner try some sliced fruit with cottage cheese. Dinner is fish, rice, salad with a healthy dressing, and your favorite fruit.

Eat before you are hungry, drink before you are thirsty. Keep those upper-body muscles firm and full. Never let yourself go more than a couple of hours without sustenance. If you don't eat now, you may eat too much later.

Regular snacks between meals assure that your system won't cannibalize your hard-earned upper body. A perfect snack is a combination of carbs and protein. Your favorite fruit and cottage cheese or peanut butter and a banana are good choices.

Spend a few minutes each evening planning the next day's meals and snacks. Examine your schedule. Figure out when you get hungry. Have appropriate snacks available. Carry a cooler in your car filled with plastic containers of your favorite foods. Pack peanut butter on whole-wheat bread, yogurt and a banana, pita bread with hummus, baby carrots, and a green pepper. Keep your desk drawer stocked with cereal bars, pretzels, dried fruit, dried soups, and oatmeal.

In Other Words

Simple carbs that have a high glycemic index travel from your stomach to your bloodstream to your muscles, liver, or fat stores very quickly.

Special-order at restaurants. Ask that your foods be poached, grilled, steamed, or baked. Request that the chef not add extra oil, cream, or butter in your dishes. Some "special sauces" are very high in calories. Remember to order dressing on the side, so *you* control how much you get.

What if you need to eat 2,000 calories a day to maintain your metabolism? It's 10:00 p.m. and so far you have only eaten 1,500 calories. Should you go to bed hungry, or eat 500 more calories?

The answer is: Don't go to bed hungry. Schedule a reasonable, 500-calorie mini-meal to ensure that your upper-body muscles stay nourished.

Making the Most of Your Meals

Your body digests and processes the food you eat, so there is a slight increase in your caloric expenditure during mealtime. It seems counter-intuitive, but while you are chowing down, you are actually leaning out your upper body. If you already graze on five or six meals a day, don't stop.

Get It Right

Eat slow-release carbs such as oatmeal and fruits and veggies with the skin. These long-chain carbs stay with you longer and provide you with much-needed vitamins, minerals, and fiber.

Fueling your workout is a major part of seeing great definition in your upper body. Eat to energize your upper body for your workouts. What you eat today and tomorrow will benefit your chest and arm workouts the next day, and the next.

Balancing your meals energizes your workouts. The quantity of food that you eat before and after your workout depends on your metabolism and your activity. You may burn between 300 and 500 calories per training session. Therefore, be sure you are eating enough to maintain your hard-earned muscle. Eat four carbs to one protein as soon after your upper-body workout as you can to speed nutrients to your depleted muscles.

And eat real food! You don't need to buy expensive supplements, and supplements don't make up for poor eating habits. Fruits and vegetables offer far more than just vitamins. Plan your meals in advance so you get all of the muscle-toning nutrients from your diet that you need.

Eat to Starve Your Fat Cells

If you don't eat enough your metabolism slows and your body holds onto your fat stores. If you eat too much, you add extra insulation around your brand new upper-body muscles.

To inspire you to stay with your eating program, pinch the fat on the back of your upper arm. Grab an inch of fat between your thumb and index finger and then decide if you really need to eat. Or, decide if the food you are about to eat will fuel your muscle or add to your fat stores.

Eating perfectly all of the time is no fun. Fortunately, no one expects you to be perfect. "Keep progressing, not perfecting" is the mantra of this program. This program has nothing to do with willpower; it just requires some thought and planning. Plan your meals in advance and have the discipline to eat every few hours.

You may benefit from a food diary to keep you on track. This is a great tool to figure out what changes you need to make to your lifestyle so it will work for you. Write down when and how much you ate. Soon you will eat every few hours and bingeing will be something other people do.

You'll know when you lose that extra fat. You'll feel better. Don't worry about what the scale says. Instead, focus on how your clothes fit. You won't be afraid to wear sleeveless shirts. When your shirts fit looser and your energy levels increase, you are on the program for life.

Your Total Program

In This Chapter

- Learn how to split your workouts up
- Pushing days, pulling days
- Cardio + Strength = Definition
- Weights work
- Beach muscle blowout

If getting a defined upper body meant spending a couple of hours a day working out, more people would have a great upper body. It's not just about working out.

To get the upper body you want, put it all together: eat right, do some easy activity, and do isolation exercises to broaden your chest and back, streamline your arms, and define your shoulders.

Eating right and general activity is the way to chisel your upper body. There is no way that you can lose fat in one certain spot unless you undergo liposuction. Doing rep after rep of push-ups won't make the backs of your arms thinner. You lose fat from your whole body. Doing push-ups, lat pull-downs, and shoulder presses will make your muscles larger. But to get that sleek, defined look, watch what you eat and include some easy activity into your program.

You will see results fast if you combine all three aspects of the program. A few minutes of easy activity, upper-body toning, and food preparation is all it takes.

And it's not that hard. The hardest part of the workout is turning off that computer. Finding the time to work out is an art. A few minutes of exercise, several times a day, boosts energy, decreases stress, builds confidence, and helps you sleep better. So if you can sneak five minutes several times a day, you will get more of your computer work done in a shorter period.

Increase Your Activity

Just move. Once you start moving it becomes a habit. Soon it will feel excruciating to sit for long periods. Your body loves to move, so let it!

No exercise gizmo is better than simply moving your body against gravity. Move at different angles and intensities to burn more calories.

Listen to your body. Talk with your physician about any tweaks or creaks that last more than a week. Stay below the symptoms of any discomfort or pain.

Move 20 minutes extra each day.

If you can work your way up to moving an extra 20 minutes each day, you are *guaranteed* to make progress. You don't have to move fast, just move.

Do all of the activities that you have been told to do to lose weight, such as taking the stairs instead of the elevator and parking in the space furthest from your office. Make your life one mini-workout after another instead of finding ways to sit.

Don't work up a sweat, but move. If you have to sit, and no one is watching, punch an imaginary boxing speed bag by rolling your hands around each other above your head.

Keep track of how many extra minutes you move each day. If you haven't reached 20 extra minutes by dinnertime, go for a quick walk.

Bet You Didn't Know

A muscle cell weighs more than a fat cell, but a fat cell is almost five times larger than a muscle cell.

Add five minutes a week until you're up to an hour.

Twenty minutes of extra activity each day is your first step toward seeing better definition in your upper body. Your next step is to add five minutes of movement each week. In just eight weeks you will be moving an hour a day beyond what you were doing before. By then you will have the chiseled arms you've been hoping for.

If your boss allows you to sit on an exercise ball instead of a chair, you burn extra calories just keeping your balance. Instead of using e-mail, walk a few steps to your colleague's office and deliver the message in person.

Move Fast or Move Slow—Just Move

You burn similar calories whether you walk a mile or jog a mile, so why not take it easy? Some people think that there is something magic about running and losing weight. Walking briskly burns even more calories than a slow jog.

If you want to maintain your upper-body muscle, walk instead of run. Pounding the pavement actually breaks down your hard-earned upper body. You probably don't want the upper body of a marathon runner, so don't train like one. Too much aerobic activity breaks down muscle tissue, and you don't want that.

Stick with nonimpact activities such as stair climbing, elliptical machines, cross-country skiing, and cycling. Do the minimum amount of cardio—30 to 45 minutes, 3 or 4 days a week. When you do too much cardio, your body uses your upper-body muscle tissue for energy. So take it down a notch.

To discover if you are doing too much cardio or working out too hard, take notice of your upper-body strength levels. If you remain strong and your upper-body muscles are full and toned, you are doing fine.

> **In Other Words** _____
>
> Train according to your *perceived exertion*. Perceived exertion is a measure of how hard you are training based on how you feel.

Accessories Make the Workout

Take a look at your shoes before you begin. Don't wear your old tennis shoes. Purchase a shoe that supports the type of activity you choose. Since you want to avoid impact activities, get a good, supportive walking shoe for the trails or treadmills. A walking shoe is specially designed with added flexibility in the ball of the foot to "toe-off" on each step.

A cross-training shoe will be fine for pedaling, stepping, or gliding. Once you find a pair you like, buy an identical pair for the office. Then over your lunch break, you can walk up the stairs of your office building and take the elevator down for a non-impact workout. Also, wear comfortable, breatheable clothing according to climate and activity.

Put Yourself in the Mood

Training your upper body in the weight room requires concentration. If you zone out during your weight workouts, you won't achieve the upper body of your dreams. But your mental state for easy activity is a different story. Movement is a mood-improver, and even just walking will lift your spirits. If you don't enjoy being alone with your thoughts, take a Walkman on your walk. Listen to talk shows or the news, or get pumped up with your favorite tunes. But don't let the music inspire you to a level of activity that breaks down your precious muscle tissue.

Working Out in Intervals

After your upper-body–toning workout, your metabolism stays revved for several minutes. The same is true after you complete your cardio workout.

In Other Words

Excess post-exercise oxygen consumption (EPOC) is the afterburn—the extra amount of calories your body continues to burn after you have completed your workout.

Interval training is a way to burn calories fast. And if you burn a lot of calories, you lose a lot of fat. On all of these interval activity programs, stay below the level of huffing and puffing and burning. Warm up for five minutes before you begin and cool down for five minutes at the completion of your workout.

If you reside near a track, try this interval recipe. After your warm-up, walk the length of the track briskly at 70 percent of your maximum effort. Walk slowly around the curve. Do this for 5 cycles. Be sure to cool down with some slow walking and easy stretching when you have completed your workout.

Here are a couple of other programs to change up your workouts and keep you progressing. Begin with easy movement, then gradually step it up. Moving fast simply means moving at a pace that is challenging but doable.

Program 1: Begin with a 5-minute warm-up of easy movement and always finish up with a 5-minute cool-down. During Week One, move for 25 minutes doing a 3-minute fast interval and a 1-minute slow interval. Week Two: Move for 30 minutes doing a 4-minute fast interval and a 1-minute slow interval.

Program 2: Recreational intervals are fun. You speed up and slow down depending on how you feel. If you're ready to pick up the pace, go for it. If you are breathless, slow down. Although recreational intervals are not structured, the benefits are the same as regular intervals.

Interval training is not magic. If you love doing intervals, have at it. If not, stay with your favorite easy activity.

Upper-Body Training

You can perform your isolation training at home, in your office, or in the gym. Train your upper-body muscles no more than twice a week, but with at least 48 hours rest in between upper-body workouts. Your exercises should take no longer than a few minutes.

How hard you train your muscles is more important than how long. Go for the burn occasionally, but if your muscles feel uncomfortable for a couple of days afterward, you went too far.

Your Personal Trainer

Choose the upper-body routine that works for you. Push one day, pull the next. Or try chest, back, and shoulders one day and arms the next day. When you stop making progress, it's time to change your program.

Find what works for you.

If you prefer to minimize your upper-body workout time, just train your entire upper body twice a week. But if you love to train your upper body, you can do a split routine. A split routine means that you will train a couple of upper-body parts a day.

If you enjoy working out daily, you can train several days a week using a split routine. Perform three sets of ten repetitions of each exercise with perfect form. Your first set is a warm-up and your second and third sets are working sets.

On Mondays do pushing exercises by working your chest with bench presses and the backs of your arms with triceps extensions.

On Wednesdays do pulling exercises by training your back with lat pull-downs and the fronts of your arms with biceps curls.

On Fridays work your shoulders with shoulder presses, lateral raises, front raises, and rear deltoid raises.

This is just one example of a split routine. Do whatever works for you. Target each muscle with a specific exercise once, or a maximum of twice, a week.

Mix and match. Your upper-body muscles need to be challenged from different angles and intensities for them to grow. Use perfect form to maximize your progress and minimize soreness.

If you are extremely short on time at home or in the gym, do supersets. This method works antagonist muscles—the front and the back of your upper body. This routine keeps your heart rate up so that your muscles get toned and streamlined simultaneously.

Perform a set of ten reps of the bench press for your chest. Without any rest, perform a set of ten reps of seated rowing for your back muscles. Continue this cycle until you have completed three sets of ten reps on both the bench press and seated rowing. By now you might need a breather, so take a one-minute break and a sip of water.

Do a set of reverse curls for the fronts of your arms. Then, without any rest do a set of close grip push-ups for your triceps. Continue this cycle so that when you are finished you have performed three sets of ten reps of both reverse curls and close grip push-ups.

And there you have it—an upper body pump in less than ten minutes (and that includes your one-minute break).

Add two reps to your program each week.

When you first begin training, your upper body responds to almost any exercise you do, especially women. Many women have never trained their upper bodies before. Once they begin training, they improve at least as fast as men.

But if you don't challenge your muscles, they stay the same. That is why you should add weight when you can complete ten repetitions with perfect form. Look for visible results in a few weeks.

Add one new isolation exercise each month.

Just as you get bored doing the same exercises, your upper-body muscles do, too. When you don't add anything new to your upper-body–isolation program, don't expect to see improvement. Adding one new exercise each month will ignite your progress.

Get It Right

Do not stretch your working muscles vigorously between sets. Wait to stretch until after the workout. Instead, use that time to mentally prepare for your next set.

Eating program

Miracle diets return every seven years with different names. The Atkins low-carb diet is similar to Dr. Stillman's diet in the 1960s, which required you to eat meat, cheese, and eggs.

Liquid diets have come and gone and so have the single food (grapefruit, cabbage) all-you-can-eat plans.

There is no doubt that you can lose weight on diets that limit you to a few food groups, but you cannot keep the weight off. So get back to the basics and do it right. Make eating right part of your lifestyle instead of "going on a diet."

Eat a balanced breakfast every morning.

Eat a substantial breakfast and it will power your workout and energize your day.

Whatever food you don't use for energy is stored in your muscles, liver, or in your fat cells.

Subtract 250 calories more each day from your diet and in a week you will lose half a pound. I know that doesn't sound like much, but use another 250 calories in exercise and you can lose about two pounds of flab in a week!

Eat a protein/carbohydrate snack after your workout.

Below is a partial list of foods on our eating program. This is just a quick sample. You may prefer emu (lean protein), kashi (complex carb), and kiwi (fruit). It really depends on your taste.

Mix and match a lean protein, complex carbohydrate, and fruit for each meal and snack throughout the day.

Sample Foods on the Eating Program

	Lean Protein	Complex Carbs	Fruit
❏	Turkey	Cruciferous Veggies	Strawberries
❏	Pork Loin	Cereals	Blueberries
❏	Dairy	Whole Grains	Raspberries
❏	Buffalo	Lentils	Pineapple

Drink water before, during, and after your workout.

Water does not provide energy, but it is involved in just about every process in the human body. Eight glasses of water a day are enough for sedentary couch potatoes, but not for you.

Drink about one milliliter of water per calorie that you burn. That means if you burn 2,000 calories working out, you need to drink an additional two liters of water.

Eat half a gram of carbohydrate per pound of body weight within 3 hours of your workout. If you weigh 150 pounds, you should eat a quick 75 grams of carbohydrate (1 banana) and 19 grams of protein (2 cups of non-fat milk). Eat to fuel your muscles. After you work out, you should eat a 4/1 ratio of carbs to protein as soon as possible to replenish glycogen stores and rebuild muscle. Not only will you feel better, you will have more energy and your arms will thank you.

Essential, Omega-Three Fats

Omega-three fats from fish and unsaturated fat from oils are part of an upper-body toning diet.

Eat dietary fat as 15 to 20 percent of your total calories. For men that is about 60 grams of fat on a 2500-calorie diet. Women should take in about 40 grams of fat on a 2000-calorie diet. Your activity level helps determine the amount of calories and fat to consume.

This eating program is your dream come true. You eat before you are hungry and you drink a lot of water throughout the day. Never let yourself go more than a few hours without food. Choose foods that you love. There are no forbidden foods; you eat what you like in moderation. Pre-prepare your foods in advance so that you know what you are going to eat tomorrow.

Feed your workouts with a combination of lean protein, starchy carbohydrates, and fibrous vegetables. When in doubt choose whole foods, natural, God-given fruits and vegetables instead of man-made, processed hydrogenated products.

Take a day off from the program once a week—that is part of the program. You never fall off the wagon, you just make better choices for your next meal.

Reading, Viewing, Surfing

Upper-body workouts are constantly changing thanks to new technology, better equipment, and innovative ideas. Keep pace with the latest fitness toys, tools, and news in these great magazines, dvd/videos, and websites.

Magazines to Motivate Your Upper-Body Workout

Magazines can provide you with the latest buzz on your upper-body training. But be careful. Sometimes the latest information presented in magazines may be tied to a product they are selling in an adjacent ad. But at least you can look at the pictures for inspiration.

Muscle and Fitness

Flex magazine

Muscle and Fitness Hers

Health

Ironman magazine

Men's Health

Natural Bodybuilding magazine

Women's Health

Videos to Change Up Your Upper-Body Routine

If you enjoy training to videos and DVDs, go for it. Once you learn the movements, adjust the weights and reps to your specific upper-body routine. I hope you enjoy some of these videos. Take away as much information from the videos as possible, regardless of whether the video personality gets on your nerves.

The Firm: Body Sculpting System 2—Upper Body Sculpt

Gilad's Quick Fit Shoulders & Arms

Gilad's Quick Fit Chest & Back

Leslie Sansone's Short Cuts Upper Body

The Firm: Upper Body Split

Cory Everson's Get Hard Arms & Shoulders

Videos and DVDs are available at Collage Video, 5390 Main St. NE, Minneapolis, MN 55421. 1-800-433-6769. www.collagevideo.com.

Websites to Bolster Your Workout

If you're computer savvy, you can find just about anything you need to know in the world of upper-body training. Here are some websites to get you started.

Food and Nutrition Information Center
www.nal.usda.gov/fnic/index.html

National Strength and Conditioning Association
www.nsca-lift.org

NetSweat.com. The Internet's Fitness Resource
www.netsweat.com

Cooper Institute
www.cooperaerobics.com

Tom Seabourne's website
www.tomseabourne.com

Index